Evelyn Carr

TOP 19 AMAZING NATURAL HOME REMEDIES TO CURE TOOTHACHE

i

Copyright @ 2023 by Evelyn Carr

All rights reserved

No part of this book may be used or reproduced by any means, graphical, electronical or mechanical, including photocopying, recording, taping or by any information storage retrieval system without the written permission of the publisher and author.

TABLE OF CONTENTS

CHAPTER ONE: Introduction

CHAPTER TWO

Evelyn Carr

CHAPTER SEVEN: Conclusion

Summary of home remedies and prevention tips — 90

CHAPTER ONE

MEANING OF TOOTHACHE

Toothache is the aggravation or irritation in or around the tooth, frequently brought about by tooth rot or contamination. It can be a moderate or severe pain in or around your jaws and teeth. It could mean that there is a problem with your gums or teeth.

CAUSES OF TOOTHACHE

Toothache can be brought on by:
- A broken tooth
- Diseased tooth
- An abscessed tooth
- A decayed filling
- Infected gums
- A poorly installed crown or filling, or a fractured tooth.

Consequently, toothache can have causes that aren't due to underlying disease Some examples are:

- Biting hard into something.
- Flossing.
- Getting something caught between braces or teeth.
- Chilled drinks or foods
- Grinding and clenching while asleep
- It can also be a normal part of a child's development (in children)

When the innermost layer of the tooth, known as the dental pulp, becomes inflamed, toothache can also occur.
Sensitive nerves and blood vessels make up the pulp.

Tooth decay causes the hard surface of the tooth to develop holes (cavities).

SYMPTOMS OF TOOTHACHE

- Gum swelling
- Abnormally red gums
- Foul-tasting discharge
- Ache
- Fever
- Difficulty in breathing or swallowing
- Headaches
- Pain
- Chills

CHAPTER TWO

COMMON DENTAL INFECTIONS THAT CAN BE PREVENTED OR CURED AT HOME WITH HOME REMEDIES

Dental infections can be stressful and worrying, especially if you are unsure of which treatment to choose. As a result, to give you an idea, a few of the most common dental infections that can be treated with home remedies are listed below.

1. Caries: Dental caries or cavities are openings caused because of tooth rot. Although they are a part of nature, infected bacteria can even affect the nerve and cause unbearable pain.

2. Disease of the gums/ Periodontal disease: They are a collective term for conditions brought on by prolonged untreated gingivitis. It then develops into periodontitis; it can likewise arrive at the jaw

bone when permitted to
progress.

3. Trauma: A tooth is more
   susceptible to bacterial
   invasion when it has
   been chipped or broken
   by an unidentified trauma.

Therefore, be prepared with
their alternative home
remedies the next time you
come across any of these
infections.

CHAPTER THREE

HOME SOLUTIONS FOR TOOTHACHE

1. ICE PACK

2. CLOVE OIL

3. TUMERIC

4. WHEATGRASS

5. SALT WATER FLUSH

6. GARLIC

7. PEPPERMINT TEA PACKS/PEPPERMINT REJUVENATING OIL

8. THYME

9. VANILLA CONCENTRATE

10. HYDROGEN PEROXIDE FLUSH

11. GUAVA LEAVES

12. TOOTHACHE PLANT

13. CAYENNE PEPPER

14. NATURAL/HERBAL TEA

15. CUCUMBER

16. CRUDE ONIONS

17. GINGER

18. VITAMIN K2 RICH OIL TO THE TOOTH

19. TOOTHPASTE

1.

1. ICE PACK

An ice pack is like a cold compress which can be used to ease any aggravation/pain you're encountering, especially when any sort of injury has caused your toothache.

At the point when you apply an ice pack, it makes the veins in the space choke. This makes torment less serious and likewise lessen any expanding and aggravation.

INSTRUCTIONS TO UTILIZE

To utilize this, wrap an ice block in a towel and hold to the impacted region for 20 minutes straight, you can repeat this at regular intervals. Additionally, you can apply the ice pack to your face.
If by any chance, you have an irritated tooth, your face could seem enlarged and puffy. If so, you can apply an ice pack to your cheek. The cool idea of the ice will decrease its expansion. Keep in mind that if your face is enlarged, you could have a serious contamination, you could even have a sore. If so, you

should talk to your dental specialist quickly. The person can exhort you on additional treatment.

2. CLOVE OIL

Clove has been very well used to treat toothaches from the beginning of time. It isn't just used as a heavenly expansion to baking and curries, it is likewise great for facilitating torment. The oil can really numb the agony and lessen irritation. Cloves contain areas of strength called eugenol, which is a characteristic germ-free and a sedative. This implies that it numbs the nerves, and furthermore forestalls further contamination.

INSTRUCTIONS TO UTILIZE

To utilize this, weaken clove oil with a transporter oil, similar to sunflower or jojoba oil. Add a proportion of around 15 drops of clove oil into one ounce of transporter oil, then spot a limited quantity of the weakened oil onto a cotton ball and apply it to the impacted region a couple of times each day.
On the other hand, you can simply add a drop of clove oil to a little glass of water and make a mouthwash.

3. TUMERIC

Tumeric, an individual from the ginger plant family is perhaps one of the most beneficial and effective plant on earth, It has an entire series of purposes and advantages. It is regularly used as a cooking flavor and a therapeutic substance in numerous normal recuperating customs. Recently, there have been a bunch of new learns about turmeric's ability and efficiency in treating dental issues and assisting with the teeth upkeep.

Turmeric is known to have cell reinforcements. It's

additionally known for its capacity to bring calming against microbial effects, be hostile to cancer-causing agents, possess antimutagenic mending characteristics to various clinical circumstances as well as to dental consideration. Turmeric has been utilized for a wide assortment of clinical circumstances.

Turmeric likewise contains a compound called curcumin, which is antibacterial, germicide, and pain relieving (torment easing). Curcumin can assist with halting your tooth torment and forestalling diseases and abscesses.

Tumeric can:

- help joints
- identify plaque
- treat the stomach related framework
- assist with getting worms out of body
- lighten gas
- assist with giving alleviation from dental torment
- ease menstrual issues
- lower cholesterol
- help dispose gallstones
- sanitize cuts, wounds, and burns
- relieve skin contaminations

- prevent cavities:
Turmeric has been
demonstrated to lower
the amount of cavity-
causing bacteria, thereby
aiding in cavity
prevention. Pit and
fissure sealants are a
protective technique
used to prevent cavities.
When turmeric is used in
conjunction with these
sealants, it has proven to
be a highly successful
cavity treatment.

- In addition to its dental
benefits, turmeric can
also assist with mental
health concerns such as
depression and anxiety.

- It alleviate infections and purify the liver.

- Reduce inflammation. Many dental issues e.g the periodontal disease and gingivitis can cause inflammation. Gingivitis is a type of gum disease that causes gum redness and irritation while Periodontal disease, which is also known as gum disease or periodontitis is when the mouth's soft tissue becomes infected and gets inflamed.
- Help reduce the symptoms and presence of premalignant sores,

wounds and lesions. In this case, you'll have to use more concentrated tumeric in more higher dose.

- Helps lessen Recurrent Aphthous Stomatitis (RAS) symptoms. RAS is an inflammatory issue where there is a constant painful mouth ulcers. These ulcers often heal and reappear very quickly, they usually come and go suddenly. Turmeric is a remedy known to help alleviate the symptoms and pain of these ulcers.

STEP BY STEP INSTRUCTIONS TO UTILIZE

You can squash tumeric to make a glue and apply to impacted region.

On the other hand, you can add a teaspoon of turmeric powder into a limited quantity of water. Add a portion of this glue to a cotton ball, and apply it directly to your irritated tooth or use as mouthwash. You might blend this glue in with honey to further develop taste.

4. SALT WATER FLUSH

An ordinary salt water wash and cold pack application can just as well cure minor disturbance. Making a salt water flush is an effective method for disinfecting your mouth. This saline blend is a disinfectant, and that implies that it keeps microscopic organisms from developing.

For some individuals, a saltwater flush is a compelling first-line treatment. Salt water is a characteristic sanitizer, and it can assist with slackening food particles and food debris that might be stuck in between your teeth.

Treating a toothache with salt water can likewise assist with decreasing irritation and mend any oral injuries.

INSTRUCTIONS TO UTILIZE

Keeping your mouth clean will assist with forestalling disease. Salt water flush can lessen how much pain you feel. Wash your mouth after every meal, when you wake up and before you go to bed. To utilize this methodology, blend half teaspoon of salt into a glass of warm water and use it as a mouthwash.

5. WHEATGRASS

Wheatgrass has innumerable recuperating, mitigating and helping properties. It contains numerous supplements, including a high chlorophyll content that assist in battling microscopic organisms.

STEP BY STEP INSTRUCTIONS TO UTILIZE

You can boil wheatgrass in a pot of water and drink or use it as a mouthwash.

6. GARLIC

For millennium, garlic has been recognized and used for its restorative properties. It doesn't just make food tasty but also assist with facilitating the aggravation of a toothache. It is also filled with antibacterial properties. Besides the fact that it can eliminate unsafe microscopic organisms that cause dental plaque, it can likewise go about as a painkiller.

At the point when you smash garlic cloves, they discharge allicin. This is a characteristic antibacterial specialist, which can help you with your tooth torment.

INSTRUCTIONS TO UTILIZE

To use garlic on a toothache, grind a garlic clove to make a glue and apply it to the impacted region. You might wish to add a smidgen of salt. On the other hand, you can slowly bite and chew a clove of new garlic or wash your mouth with garlic water. All things considered, you might need to circle back to some pepppermint!

7. PEPPERMINT TEA PACKS/PEPPERMINT REJUVENATING OIL

Both can be utilized to numb pain/agony and mitigate delicate gums.

Peppermint includes menthol, a functioning fixing that is solid enemy of bacterial properties. These properties may likewise assist with easing your tooth torment normally. Like an additional benefit, peppermint will give you a minty new breath!

STEP BY STEP INSTRUCTIONS TO UTILIZE

Permit a pre-owned tea pack to chill off a little prior to applying it to the impacted region. It ought to, in any case be somewhat warm.
You can likewise use this technique to cool the region instead of warm it.
To do this, put a pre-owned tea pack in the cooler for two or three minutes to chill it and afterward apply the pack to your tooth.
On the other hand, you can pour little amount of peppermint oil in a cotton wool and apply on impacted region.

8. THYME

(THYME OIL, TEA OR NEW THYME LEAVES)

Thyme is an extraordinary spice to use in cooking. It is filled with a strong cell reinforcement, antimicrobial and antibacterial properties that can as well assist with treating toothaches. Thyme is brimming with thymol, an antifungal and germ-less dynamic fixing. This can make it an extraordinary medicinal ointment for tooth aches and contaminations, It even helps battle microbes that support tooth rot.

STEP BY STEP INSTRUCTIONS TO UTILIZE

To utilize this, weaken thyme natural oil with a transporter oil, and afterward apply it to the impacted region.
You can likewise add a drop of the oil to a little glass of water and make a mouthwash.
On the other hand, you can add the natural thyme oil directly to the affected gums and teeth.
You can likewise taste thyme tea or bite new thyme leaves. Thyme leaves are tiny, so it is really smart to bite them on the opposite side of your

irritated tooth because if the little leaves get into the contaminated/affected region, it could lead to additional issues.

9. VANILLA CONCENTRATE

Vanilla concentrate contains liquor, which can help make painful sores less sensitive. Its demonstrated cancer prevention agent properties additionally make it a powerful healer. However, make sure you use the authentic and unadulterated vanilla instead of the impersonated or adulterated one.

INSTRUCTIONS TO UTILIZE

To utilize this, pour a moderate quantity of vanilla concentrate on a cotton ball or your finger and apply it to

the affected region a couple
of times each day.

10. HYDROGEN PEROXIDE FLUSH

A hydrogen peroxide wash may likewise assist with easing torment and irritation. As well as killing micro-organisms, hydrogen peroxide can lessen plaque and mend draining gums.

THE MOST EFFECTIVE METHOD TO UTILIZE

Ensure that you properly weaken the hydrogen peroxide by pouring a small amount of hydrogen peroxide into equal amount of water,

Evelyn Carr

and use it as a mouthwash.
Try not to swallow it.

11. GUAVA LEAVES

Guava leaves have mitigating properties that can assist with recuperating wounds. They likewise have antimicrobial action that can support oral consideration.

STEP BY STEP INSTRUCTIONS TO UTILIZE

To utilize this cure, bite on new guava leaves or add squashed guava paste into bubbling water to make a mouthwash.

12. TOOTHACHE PLANT

The suitably named toothache plant is a blooming plant that fills in tropical and subtropical districts. Its dynamic compound, spilanthol, has calming properties, as indicated by a 2021 survey. It likewise gives a desensitizing sensation when bitten.
However this plant is by and large thought to be protected, you shouldn't utilize it if:
- You're sensitive to plants in the daisy family
- You drink liquor
- You use diuretics

- You have prostate
  disease
- You're pregnant.

13. CAYENNE PEPPER

Cayenne pepper might be a typical flavor used in dishes all over the planet It might look odd attempting to involve this kind of pepper as a relief from discomfort, notwithstanding, you'll be stunned that this pepper can make all the difference. Cayenne pepper contains a part called capsaicin, which can impede torment signs to the cerebrum and normally diminish torment. While it can be consumed whole, you can blend cayenne flavor in with water and apply it to the tooth

for decreasing irritation until
you get to a dental specialist.

14. NATURAL/HERBAL TEA

Home grown teas are some other dependable cure if you have any desire to dispose off enlarged gums, among different diseases. Curiously, establishing that particular plant in your nursery could give you an eternity supply of this tea. Or on the other hand, you could purchase the leaves and stem of these spices and put them in steaming hot water to set up some tea.
Fenugreek and Goldenseal are the two best and sound decisions for tea as they

assist with mitigating any side effect of a tooth contamination. Moreover, both the plants have insusceptibility supporting anti-toxin properties and can be found effectively across supermarkets.

STEP BY STEP INSTRUCTIONS TO UTILIZE

Attempt this enlarged gums home cure by blending your tea packs in warm water and drinking something like three cups day to day. This will assist you with taking out the most honed gum torment.

15. CUCUMBER

You may definitely be aware of cucumber's mitigating impacts. This is the motivation behind why such countless individuals use it as a solution for puffy eyes. It has anti-hemostatic properties, and that implies that it assists with keeping blood inside a vein.

STEP BY STEP INSTRUCTIONS TO UTILIZE

To utilize cucumber on your tooth torment, cut a piece and hold it to the impacted region.

You can likewise make a
combination of cucumber and
ocean salt and use it as a
glue on the tooth.
Is your cucumber In the
cooler? Bring it up to room
temperature prior to applying
it to your delicate teeth.

16. CRUDE ONIONS

Onions are scrumptious expansion to food, however did you have any idea that onions are disinfectants? Yes, it's true! They are loaded with antimicrobial properties. This can assist crude onions with killing the microscopic organisms in your mouth and lessen your aggravation.

TO UTILIZE;

Put a crude onion on the impacted regin. It could make your eyes water, yet dental specialists concur that it will

probably assist with dulling
the aggravation.

17. GINGER

Ginger is a strong clean plant, and it tastes perfect. New ginger is loaded with dynamic fixings. These includes zingerones, shogaols, and gingerols. Biting crude ginger is an extraordinary method for decreasing specific microscopic organisms in your mouth.
Lessening specific microbes can assist with torment and can stop further contamination. As well as biting on crude ginger, you can add new ginger to your

food. It has incredible
advantages and tastes
delightful.

18. APPLY A NUTRIENT K2 RICH OIL TO THE TOOTH

Your body has nutrient K2 subordinate proteins that are set free from the dental mash to battle tooth aggravation called osteocalcin. Eating an eating routine with a lot of nutrient K2 rich food varieties might assist with battling toothaches normally.

19. TOOTHPASTE

Frequently when our lacquer separates, our teeth become touchy, which can cause agony and pain. Picking the right toothpaste can assist with combatting this issue, as well as brushing daintily to guarantee not to harm the gums.
Turmeric toothpaste can lessen plaque and irritation. It very well may be utilized to both treat and forestall aggravation.

One more incredible treatment for periodontitis and gum disease is using a glue made from the combination of salt and mustard oil.

~~

The above tips can regularly cure minor torment and disturbance, however more serious toothaches might require a dental specialist's intercession.
You should see your dental specialist if the side effects continue for over a little while so they can direct you on the best way to ease your side effects and forestall future pain.

You ought to likewise converse with your dental

specialist prior to utilizing any of the accompanying cures assuming you're pregnant, breastfeeding, or have any ailment that might be influenced by natural fixings. You can do the accompanying cures at home, however you might have to source the fixings from your neighborhood wellbeing food store or on the web.

Your mouth, teeth, and gums are reasonable delicate as of now, so buying these fixings from a respectable manufacturer is particularly significant. This can lessen your gamble of possible bothering.

CHAPTER FOUR

OTHER TIPS TO ASSUAGE TOOTHACHE

Assuming you have any issues where you have a toothache around evening time and you couldn't alleviate it with some of the above home cures maybe because they weren't available at the moment or because of any other reasons, you can quickly try to reduce the pain/aggravation by:

- Washing with fluoride mouthwash

- Washing with salt water
- Utilizing a desensitizing gel
- Applying an ice pack
- In order to reduce expansion and keep blood from pooling or gathering together in your cheek, you can try laying down with your face up.

- You can likewise ingest mitigating medications like ibuprofen, Advil, Motrin or naproxen. They function effectively against dental agony since they lessen irritation. Ongoing information has shown that the mixture of Advil (ibuprofen) and Tylenol (acetaminophen) exist as powerful narcotics for tooth yet it's advisable to limit the usage of drugs containing benzocaine.

- Flossing and brushing gently however consistently can assist with eliminating disturbing food particles and assist with lessening toothache.

- You can make a strong, effective mouthwash by bubbling turmeric powder, cloves, guava leaves, and water together. This mouthwash can assist with lessening

aggravation, pain,
irritation and agony as
well as assisting with
treating gum disease and
periodontal sickness.
Make a point to allow the
blend to cool before you
use it.

CHAPTER FIVE

PREVENTION TIPS FOR TOOTHACHE
HOW CAN TOOTHACHES BE FORESTALLED?

Toothache can be forestalled/prevented through the following ways:

- Following great oral cleaning practices
- Flossing and Brushing routinely with fluoride-containing toothpaste
- Flushing a few times per day with a germ-free mouthwash

- Limiting the consumption of sweet and acidic food varieties and beverages
- A few food sources which can particularly cause plaque development include:

-Citrus
-Bread
-Acrid confections
-Potato chips
-Dried organic products
-Carbonated drinks
-Liquor
-Ice

- Brushing and washing teeth after eating any of these food varieties or limiting them in one's diet can assist with preventing plaque development.

- Visiting the dental specialist consistently (in any event, two times per year)
- Utilizing a mouthguard for teeth crushing

CHAPTER SIX

WHEN TO SEE / CALL A DENTAL SPECIALIST

In a situation whereby your toothache is extreme or is the consequence of a more serious ailment, it is important that you receive immediate dental attention, see your dental specialist so you can treat it appropriately. Numerous toothaches will require clinical consideration. An over-the-counter pain killer, for example, ibuprofen could help until you see a dental specialist.

SIGNS THAT YOUR TOOTHACHE REQUIRES PROFICIENT CONSIDERATION

You ought to go to your dental specialist if:

- You have a toothache that goes for more than 1 or 2 days
- Your toothache is excruciating
- You have a fever, ear infection, or torment after opening your mouth wide

WHAT'S IN STORE DURING A DENTAL ARRANGEMENT

During your arrangement, your dental specialist will initially get your clinical history and lead an actual test. They will ask you inquiries about the ache, for example, when it began, how serious it is, where the aggravation is found, what exacerbates the aggravation, and what improves it. Your dental specialist will look at your mouth, teeth, gums, jaws, tongue, throat, sinuses, ears, nose, and neck. X-beams might be taken as well as different tests, contingent upon what your dental specialist suspects is causing your toothache.

HOW YOUR DENTAL SPECIALIST TREATS YOUR TOOTHACHE WILL RELY UPON THE REASON

1. Dental rot: In the event that a pit or dental rot is causing your toothache, your dental specialist will probably eliminate the rot and put in a filling.

2. Filling: When a hole is taken out from your tooth, your dental specialist will occupy the space with a

tooth-hued material. If by any case, the current filling is also causing you torment, they might supplant it with another filling.

3. Ulcer: Ulcer, a dental sore is a tooth contamination that can happen if, by any chance, a hole goes untreated. In case you have a sore, your dental specialist might recommend anti-toxins, play out a root waterway, or concentrate your tooth.

4. Teeth crushing (bruxism):
   If grating or grinding your
   teeth is the cause of the
   pain, your dental
   specialist might suggest
   a mouthguard.

5. Periodontal sickness:
   When plaque
   development prompts
   gum disease, it's
   workable for you to foster
   periodontal illness. This
   gum contamination
   needs your dental
   specialist to eliminate
   tartar from your teeth and
   slow sickness movement.

Furthermore, treatment for a toothache relies upon the reason. If it is a hole that is causing the toothache, your dental specialist may fill the pit or possibly extricate the tooth, if essential. A root channel may be required if the reason for the toothache is not set to be a contamination of the tooth's nerve.

If microscopic organisms that have worked their direction into the internal parts of the tooth cause such a contamination, an anti-microbial might be endorsed assuming that there is fever or enlarging of the jaw.

Evelyn Carr

SIGNIFICANCE OF LOOKING FOR PROFICIENT DENTAL CONSIDERATION WHEN FUNDAMENTAL

Dental consideration is everything with regards to the strength of your mouth, teeth, and gums. In case you want proficient assistance with your teeth, visit your nearby dental specialist in tremont for dental consideration.
Indeed, even something as straightforward as dealing with the teeth needs proficient direction. This is on the grounds that the teeth aren't

100 percent sound simply by brushing and flossing alone. Having a bad dental wellbeing will prompt pits, periodontitis, tooth rot, and gum illnesses that can be connected to the heart and different pieces of the body. Proficient dental consideration is required to guarantee a solid mouth, teeth, and gums.

FOR WHAT REASON IS DENTAL CONSIDERATION SIGNIFICANT?

Dental consideration guarantees that the teeth you have will be solid until you arrive at the ideal age when the teeth usually debilitate. This is very important in light of the fact that it is normal to lose teeth the more older you become.

.

WHY IS PROFICIENT DENTAL CONSIDERATION   REQUIRED?

Proficient dental consideration is needed even if you don't want it or think you don't really need it because experts find out about the condition of the teeth and will be more capable at assessing whether the teeth need special treatment. The following are motivations behind why proficient dental consideration is important:

1. **FORESTALLING TOOTH ROT**: Tooth rot

is something that you
can't recognize without
help from anyone else
until the aggravation
begins. Ordinary exams
could be a decent choice
since tooth rot needs
attention, and not all
could be visible.
Forestalling tooth rot is
one justification for why
you want proficient
dental consideration. You
alone can't make tooth
rot vanish definitely
because you can't work
on yourself, and some of
the time used in cleaning
your teeth isn't sufficient.

2. **EARLY LOCATION OF MOUTH ILLNESSES:** Dental consideration will help in the early location of mouth illnesses. Mouth infections are more straightforward to deal with when diagnosed before they deteriorate.

3. **FURTHER DEVELOPS TEETH WELLBEING**: At the point when your teeth are not routinely cleaned expertly, this might prompt staining which happens when you eat things that has high sugar content.

Teeth care needs proficient direction. This is on the grounds that the teeth aren't hundred percent clean and germ-free simply by brushing and flossing alone.

4. **YOUR DENTAL SPECIALIST CHECKS FOR MORE THAN CAVITIES:** Albeit, the greater part of us stress over the dental specialist finding holes, there is a great deal more that the dental specialist is checking for with an oral test. The dental specialist checks for oral cleanliness, oral

malignant growth, and early indications of gum sickness as well as searching for caries illness.

The dental specialist can make you aware of issues with dry mouth. In some cases, other ailments like oral thrush are gotten by your dental specialist, and those conditions can highlight bigger medical problems.

5. **Issues Can Be Dealt With More Successfully And Less costly Whenever Diagnosed Early:** Caries that are treated while little are

more affordable. A little dental caries might be a decent contender for remineralization treatment. Regardless of whether it answer totally to remineralization treatment, it's more affordable to treat a little depression than to allow it to develop enormously enough to require a root waterway, or more regrettable, an extraction. Early gum sickness is more straightforward to treat than laid out gum infection and is less inclined to require careful intervention.

6. **KEEPS A LOVELY GRIN**

   Keeping a lovely grin is something to take a stab at. Dental consideration will guarantee that the grins you appreciate and like putting on will be protected as far as possible.

7. **YOUR HOME CONSIDERATION ROUTINE CAN BE MORE SUCCESSFUL WITH SOME EXPERT DIRECTION**: Your home care routine is crucial to your oral wellbeing. A large portion of the hours spent really focusing on

your teeth are the ones
you spend at home as
opposed to in a dental
specialist's seat. Your
dental consideration
experts can assist you
with capitalizing on this
time in several different
ways. To begin with, they
can tell you how powerful
you are being in your
consideration.
Assuming you are
missing spots brushing
or need to clean between
teeth better, they can tell
you how to work on your
consideration. The dental
experts engaged with
your wellbeing can
likewise suggest ideal

items for your particular necessities. Assuming you are battling to clean well with floss, they can suggest other cleaning approaches like water cleaners or little, interdental brushes. They likewise can suggest oral purging items that are appropriate for your particular circumstance.

8. **YOUR ORAL WELLBEING IS ESSENTIAL FOR YOUR GENERAL WELLBEING AND OUGHT NOT BE DISREGARDED**: Gum sickness isn't the main contamination connected

to the microscopic organisms normally tracked down in an undesirable mouth. Work done by some specialists demonstrates a consistent idea between coronary illness and gum sickness — the microscopic organisms that make for undesirable oral plaques are found in plaques related with coronary illness. Notwithstanding coronary illness, different circumstances like diabetes and certain auto-resistant infections have a muddled relationship with oral wellbeing, and treating them successfully requires keeping steady over your oral wellbeing. Visit could distinguish dangerous illnesses. Bad oral wellbeing can prompt lethal circumstances, for example, respiratory failures and strokes. Preventive dental exams can assist with distinguishing conditions like oral malignant growth, which is treatable whenever identified early. Research shows that having your teeth expertly cleaned can assist with decreasing your gamble for respiratory failure and stroke. Persistent aggravation of the gums is behind this affiliation. With standard cleaning and scaling, we can decrease aggravation causing microorganisms.

9. **GIVES YOU GENUINE SERENITY**: For this reason you ought to routinely visit your dental specialist. A dental specialist will actually want to stay aware of what's happening in your mouth, help with torment and distress and afterward give you an

Evelyn Carr

arrangement for a
development.

CHAPTER SEVEN

SUMMARY

In rundown, at whatever point you have a toothache, think about utilizing these home cures.

- You can try cleaning your mouth by either flossing, brushing and flushing with salt water, mouthwash, or hydrogen peroxide and see whether that brings some help.

- You can likewise utilize an ice pack, Attempt

pressure point massage,
and bite on new garlic,
tumeric, onion or ginger.
You can make some
clove or home grown tea,
have some peppermint
or new cucumber, add a
Cayenne flavor to the
impacted tooth. Once
more you can go over
the home cures and see
the one which suits you
best. Nonetheless,
Assuming the pain is
getting too extreme,
excruciating or constant,
try to visit your dental
specialist.

Evelyn Carr

Thanks so much, dear readers!

I wish you a life free of pain and full of healthiness!

____

www.ingramcontent.com/pod-product-compliance
Lightning Source LLC
Chambersburg PA
CBHW050831260726

48660CB00006B/2174